EAT CHOCOLATE, LOSE WEIGHT!

10 Amazing Dark Chocolate

Recipes

For

Weight Loss

Candy J. Coyle

DISCLAIMER

TABLE OF CONTENTS

DARK CHOCOLATE: YOUR DELICIOUS WEIGHT-LOSS FRIEND!

DARK CHOCOLATE: YOUR DELICIOUS WEIGHT-LOSS FRIEND!

PART ONE

Chapter ONE

THE POWER OF DARK CHOCOLATE

Are you prepared to start a tasty journey towards a better way of life? We're about to enter the beautiful realm of dark chocolate, so hold on tight! Yes, you heard correctly: dark chocolate can make a wonderful ally in your efforts to lose weight.

Let's explore the techniques for adopting a healthy lifestyle while enjoying this sweet delicacy.

Imagine yourself enjoying a decadent, velvety piece of dark chocolate. As the smoothness melts on your tongue, your taste buds start to dance in ecstasy. Did you realize, though, that dark chocolate is capable of more than just tantalizing your taste buds?

It resembles a superhero in dessert form! Strong antioxidants found in dark chocolate can protect your body from bothersome free radicals.

As a result, you are providing your cells with nourishment from the inside out while indulging in its decadent flavor.

Let's now discuss things of the heart, both metaphorically and physically. The use of dark chocolate may have cardiovascular advantages. Your blood vessels can benefit from the excellent flavonoids and polyphenols found in dark chocolate by staying flexible and supporting normal blood flow.

Every time you take a bite, it's like giving your heart a tiny love letter.

But wait, we're not finished yet! Dark chocolate has a cunning way of making you feel better. When you bite into a piece of your favourite chocolate, do you ever feel complete bliss? It's science, therefore it's not just in your head!

Dark chocolate contains substances that can cause the brain's "feel-good" neurotransmitters, serotonin and endorphins, to be released. Therefore, even a small bit of dark chocolate can make you happy and your weight-loss journey much more enjoyable.

Let's now talk about portion management, the proverbial "elephant in the room." We are all aware that consuming something in excess might undermine our efforts to lose weight. But don't worry! If you take care to limit your intake, dark chocolate can still be your ally.

As tempting as it may be, enjoy a little portion of chocolate rather than a whole bar in one sitting. Consider it a daily pleasure, a brief period of unadulterated joy that won't impede your growth.

However, there's still more! The flavors of dark chocolate go well together. Combine it with nutrient-dense foods like crisp berries or juicy orange slices. Your mouth will experience a symphony of flavors as a result of the fruits' vivid hues and inherent sweetness, which work in harmony with the rich chocolate flavor.

If you're up for it, you may also add some nuts for a delicious crunch. It's the ideal balance of tastes and textures that will make your mouth water.
So, my friend, keep in mind that dark chocolate may be your ally, your confidant, and your little guilty pleasure as you set out on your weight-loss path.

Accept the magic of antioxidants, the potential cardiovascular advantages, and the mood-enhancing effects they may have. But always approach it mindfully, enjoying every bite and recognizing the happiness it offers. Enjoy that delicious dark chocolate now, because even a better way of life should allow for occasional indulgence!

Some valuable nutrients of this amazing chocolate are:

1. 604 calories
2. 7.87 g of protein
3. 43.06 g of fat
4. 46.36 g of carbohydrates
5. 11.00 g of dietary fiber
6. 24.23 g of sugar
7. 12.02 milligrams (mg) of iron
8. 230.00 mg of magnesium
9. 3.34 mg of zinc

Did you know that eating dark chocolate could fight off these?

1. Diabetes and heart disease
2. Parkinson's condition
3. Alzheimer's condition
4. Cancer
5. Eye condition

Dark chocolate consumption on a regular basis may help lower the risk of heart disease. High blood pressure and high cholesterol are two important risk factors for heart disease that are impacted by some of the components found in dark chocolate, particularly flavanols.

Chapter TWO

UNDERSTANDING WEIGHT-LOSS

We're glad you're here, weight loss world! In this chapter, we'll go deeply into the science behind losing those excess pounds and learn how to become a better, fitter version of yourself. Therefore, grab a drink of water, put on your thinking gear, and let's begin!

Calories In vs. Calories Out

Calories in minus calories out is the fundamental formula for calculating weight reduction. The fundamental idea is that in order to lose weight, you must burn more calories than you take in. This results in a calorie deficit, which forces your body to use its fat reserves as a source of energy.

Nutrition's Function

In order to lose weight, proper nutrition is essential. It involves feeding your body the correct kinds of nutrients, not just calculating calories. A range of nutrient-dense foods, such as fruits, vegetables, whole grains, lean meats, and healthy fats, are included in a well-balanced diet.

Portion Control And Mindful Eating

When it comes to controlling your calorie intake, portion control is essential. It's crucial to pay attention to portion sizes as well as your body's signals of hunger and fullness. Take your time, enjoy every bite, and pay attention to how you're feeling physically. A healthier relationship with food can be fostered and overeating can be reduced by eating consciously.

Move Your Body to Lose Weight

Not only is exercise crucial for overall health, it also helps people lose weight effectively. Regular exercise aids in calorie burning, raises metabolism, and develops lean muscular mass. Whether it's dancing, jogging, swimming, or playing a sport, choose activities that you want to do. The goal is to start moving and incorporate it into your everyday routine in a pleasurable way.

Recuperation and Rest

Although it may come as a surprise, adequate relaxation and good sleep are essential for weight loss. Your hormones might be disturbed by lack of sleep, which increases appetite and desires. To aid your body's healing process, emphasise self-care and aim for 7-9 hours of sleep each night.

Patience and Consistency

Keep in mind that lasting weight loss is a journey, not a race. It's critical to approach it patiently, consistently, and with a good outlook. Set reasonable objectives, acknowledge your accomplishments along the road, and don't let tiny setbacks derail you. Although developing healthy behaviors takes time, the benefits are worthwhile.

The Strength of Encouragement

Having a support system can significantly improve your weight loss efforts. Be in the company of inspiring and motivating individuals. Join online communities, workout classes, or if necessary, seek professional advice. You may learn from one another, share experiences, and maintain motivation by working together to accomplish your goals.

It's time to put your knowledge of the principles of weight reduction into practice now that you have a firm grasp of them. We'll examine how dark chocolate may be a delectable and useful ally on your weight loss quest in the future chapters. Stay tuned and be ready to learn about the amazing connection between chocolate and a healthy way of life!

PART TWO

Chapter THREE

ADDING DARK CHOCOLATE TO YOUR DIET

It's time to understand how to include this delicious indulgence in your regular diet now that we've established the wonderful weight-loss advantages of dark chocolate. Prepare to indulge guilt-free as we look at tasty and inventive ways to enjoy the health benefits of dark chocolate without jeopardizing your weight loss plans.

Quality Counts

Quality is important when it comes to dark chocolate. Choose bars with a high cocoa solids content, preferably 70% or more.

This makes sure you're getting the most nutritious advantages possible without consuming too much sugar or pointless chemicals.

The Key Word Is Moderation

Even though dark chocolate can help you lose weight, use restraint when eating it. Finding the ideal balance is key. Depending on how bitter the chocolate is, try to limit yourself to one or two small squares as a serving size. This lets you take advantage of the taste and advantages without consuming excessive amounts of calories.

Choose Your Snacks Wisely

Need a noon energy boost? Replace your typical sugary snacks with a dark chocolate bar. Its flavorful properties might help you fulfill cravings and stay energized all day long.

For an additional boost of nutrition and a well-balanced snack, combine it with some almonds or a piece of fruit.

Boost Your Breakfast

Add some dark chocolate to your morning ritual to get your day off to a great start. For a delicious crunch and a hint of chocolatey sweetness, top your oatmeal or yogurt with cocoa nibs or shavings. For a luxurious twist, try incorporating dark chocolate into your pancake batter or adding it to smoothies.

Desserts with a Twist

Who said eating desserts and losing weight couldn't coexist? Add some dark chocolate to your sweet desserts to add some creativity. Prepare a batch of dark chocolate avocado mousse or treat yourself to a bowl of strawberries covered in the substance.

In addition to having a delicious flavor combination, these sweets are low in calories.

Savory Surprises

Dark chocolate isn't just for people with a sweet taste. It can also give savory meals more complexity and depth. For a rich and enticing flavor, try adding a tiny bit of dark chocolate to mole or chili sauce. Your culinary explorations will be enhanced by the contrast between the savory ingredients and the bitter chocolate.

Indulgent Mindfulness

Finally, keep in mind to enjoy each meal. You may truly appreciate the experience and be in the moment when you eat mindfully. Take your time, enjoy the distinct flavors, and let the chocolate melt in your lips.

You may get the most satisfaction out of your indulgence in dark chocolate by practising mindfulness.

With these innovative suggestions, you can easily include dark chocolate in your regular diet while pursuing your weight loss objectives. Let dark chocolate be your lovely travel companion on this savory journey to a better self, and go ahead and embrace the taste.

Chapter FOUR

THE RECIPES

Pistachio and Dried Cranberry Dark Chocolate Bark

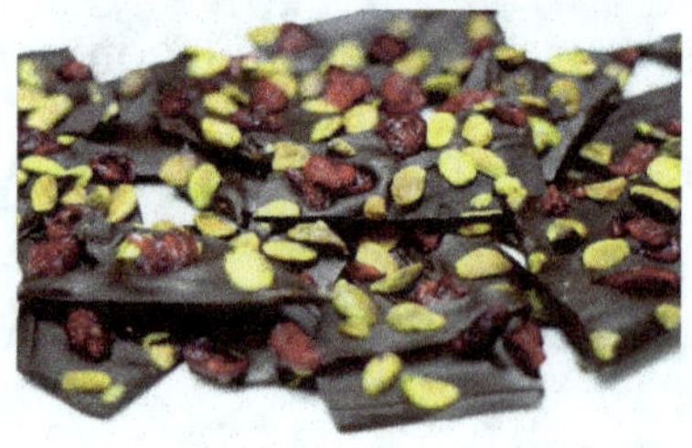

Enjoy a pleasure without feeling guilty by combining dark chocolate's health benefits with the crunch of pistachios and the tart sweetness of dried cranberries. In addition to satisfying your cravings, this delicious Dark Chocolate Bark with Pistachios and Dried Cranberries will help you achieve your weight loss objectives.

So let's get started with the recipe and learn about the advantages as we go!

Ingredients

- 8 ounces of chopped dark chocolate with at least 70% cocoa solids.
- ½ cup roughly chopped shelled pistachios
- A half cup of dried cranberries

Instructions

1. Use parchment paper or a silicone mat to line a baking sheet and set it aside.

2. Melt the dark chocolate, stirring regularly, in a heatproof bowl that can be used in the microwave or a heatproof bowl that is placed over a pan of simmering water.

3. Slather the prepared baking sheet with the melted chocolate. Spread it thinly and uniformly using a spatula.

4. Top the melted chocolate with the chopped pistachios and dried cranberries.

Make sure they attach nicely by gently pressing them into the chocolate.

5. Chill the baking sheet in the fridge for about 30 minutes, or until the chocolate is fully set.

6. Take the baking sheet out of the fridge once the chocolate has solidified. Use a knife or your hands to cut the bark into smaller, erratic pieces.

7. Plate and savour! Any residual bark should be kept in a cool, airtight container.

Weight-Loss Benefits

Let's discuss how this decadent Dark Chocolate Bark with Pistachios and Dried Cranberries will aid in your efforts to lose weight.

1. Satisfying Pistachios: Pistachios are delicious and rich in fiber, protein, and healthy fats. Together, these nutrients make you feel satisfied and full, which will help you restrain your appetite and prevent overeating.

2. Tangy Cranberries: This chocolate bark gets a taste boost from dried cranberries. These little berries include a variety of vitamins and minerals and are an excellent source of dietary fiber. Additionally, they provide a hint of natural sweetness without the need for added sugar.

This Dark Chocolate Bark, which combines the advantages of dark chocolate, pistachios, and dried cranberries, is a pleasant and nutritional treat that may be included in your weight-loss strategy. Don't forget to take it slowly and deliberately, and enjoy it in moderation.

Make this delicious Pistachio and Dried Cranberry Dark Chocolate Bark right away. It's time to indulge your cravings without jeopardizing your attempts to lose weight. Cheers to indulgence!

Dark Chocolate Peanut Butter Cups Made from Scratch

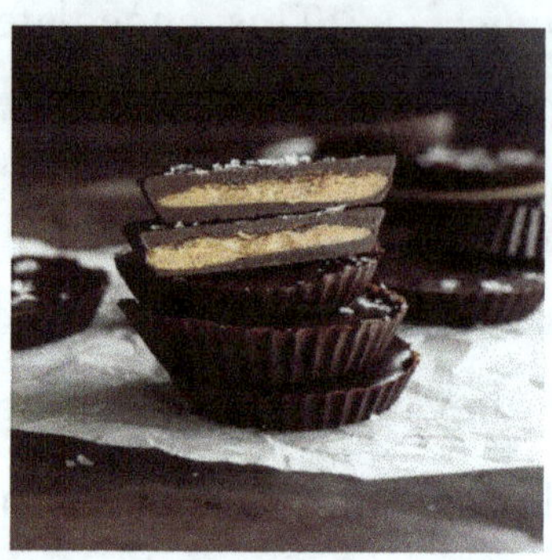

With this delicious recipe for natural dark chocolate peanut butter cups, you can indulge your sweet craving without deviating from your weight loss plans. These tiny cups of delight are proof that indulgence and weight loss are compatible.

Ingredients:

- 1 cup natural peanut butter (choose between smooth and crunchy).

- 2 tablespoons of honey or any natural sweetener of your choice

- 1 teaspoon vanilla extract

- ¼ teaspoon sea salt, if desired (for the ideal sweet-salty combination).
- 10 ounces of dark chocolate with a minimum cocoa content of 70%
- A silicone mold or muffin pan for forming the cups.
- Optional cupcake liners for simple removal

Instructions:

1. Place the natural peanut butter, honey or other preferred sweetener, vanilla extract, and sea salt (if used) in a mixing bowl. Stir everything up thoroughly until well-combined.

2. Use a double boiler or a microwave-safe bowl to liquefy half of the dark chocolate. until it's smooth and creamy, stir occasionally.

3. To make removal later on easier, line the silicone mold or muffin tin with cupcake liners.

4. Fill each cup with a little amount of melted dark chocolate and distribute it evenly across the bottom.

5. To gently harden the chocolate, place the muffin pan or mold in the refrigerator for about 10 minutes.

6. Take the tin out of the fridge and top each chocolate foundation with a liberal dollop of the peanut butter mixture, leaving a tiny gap around the borders.

7. Lightly flatten the peanut butter mixture by gently pressing it down.

8. Melt the last of the dark chocolate and drizzle it over the peanut butter, thoroughly encasing it.

9. Smooth the top layer of chocolate using a spoon or spatula to make sure the peanut butter is completely encased.

10. After chilling for at least 30 minutes, or until the chocolate is set and solid, put the muffin pan or mold back in the refrigerator.

11. After the peanut butter cups have fully hardened, remove them from the mold or pan. Peel off cupcake liners if you're using them.

12. Until you're ready to eat them, keep the natural dark chocolate peanut butter cups in the refrigerator in an airtight container.

Weight-Loss Benefits

1. The best part is that these delicious sweets not only fulfill your sweet tooth but also offer a variety of health advantages.

2. Natural peanut butter and dark chocolate combine to make a delicious flavor balance, and the dark chocolate also aids in weight loss.

3. A fantastic source of protein and healthy fats, natural peanut butter can help you feel filled for longer and support weight loss efforts.

4. Due to its high cocoa content, dark chocolate has antioxidants and fiber that help with digestion and cardiovascular health.

Therefore, enjoy these natural dark chocolate peanut butter cups guilt-free.

They are a lovely treat that aids in your efforts to lose weight and enables you to take pleasure in life's sweeter aspects.

Paleo Cashew Truffles

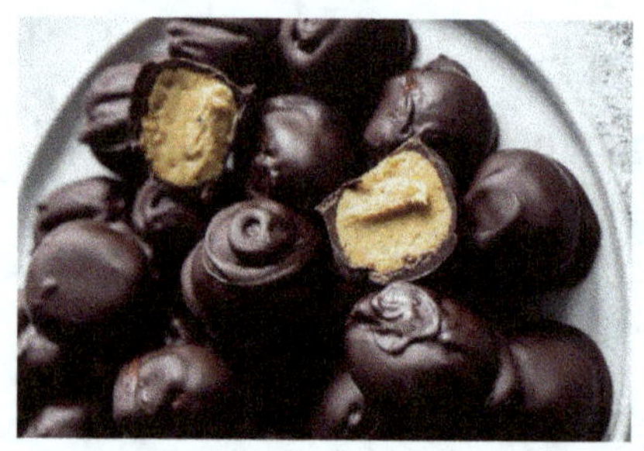

Enjoy these delectable Paleo Cashew Truffles guilt-free pleasure. These truffles will sate your sweet desire while helping you to achieve your weight loss goals because they are filled with savory tastes and healthy components. Prepare to indulge in a healthy form of chocolate ecstasy!

Ingredients:

- 1 cup uncooked cashews
- ¼ cup chocolate powder, unsweetened
- 2 teaspoons of pure maple syrup
- Optional toppings include unsweetened shredded coconut, broken almonds, or cocoa powder for rolling.
- 1 teaspoon vanilla essence
- 1 pinch sea salt

Instructions:

1. Process the raw cashews in a food processor until they resemble fine meal.

2. Fill the food processor with cocoa powder, maple syrup, vanilla essence, and a dash of sea salt. The mixture should be pulsed until it forms a sticky dough.

3. Scoop out tablespoon-sized chunks of dough and roll them between your palms to form balls.

4. To add even more flavor and texture to the truffles, if preferred, roll them in unsweetened

shredded coconut, broken almonds, or cocoa powder.

5. To firm up, place the truffles in the refrigerator for at least 30 minutes on a baking sheet coated with parchment paper.

Your Paleo Cashew Truffles are ready to eat once they have chilled! For up to a week, keep them in the refrigerator in an airtight container.

Weight Loss Benefits

You might be wondering how these delicious truffles will help you on your weight-loss journey right now. Let me tell you about their wonderful advantages:

1. Nutrient-rich Cashews: In addition to being creamy and tasty, cashews also include a range of nutrients that aid in weight loss. They provide you with a high amount of protein and beneficial fats, which can help you feel full and reduce your hunger.

2. Natural Sweetness: The truffles are slightly sweetened by using pure maple syrup rather than processed sugars.

You may fulfill your desires while avoiding the hazards of added sugars that can thwart your attempts at weight loss by choosing natural sweeteners.

3. Satisfying Treat: These Paleo Cashew Truffles are made to be an indulgent treat. The cashews' blend of fiber, protein, and healthy fats can support your weight reduction goals by helping you feel full and preventing overeating.

3. Portion Restrict: You may restrict the amount of truffles you eat by rolling them into bite-sized pieces. This enables you to monitor your intake while still indulging in a tasty pleasure. When it comes to any indulgence while trying to lose weight, keep in mind that moderation is vital.

Enjoy these Paleo Cashew Truffles without feeling guilty! They're a delicious method to sate your sweet need while continuing to work toward your weight loss objectives. Enjoy every delicious taste of chocolate while embarking on the path to a better, happier you.

Avocado Mousse

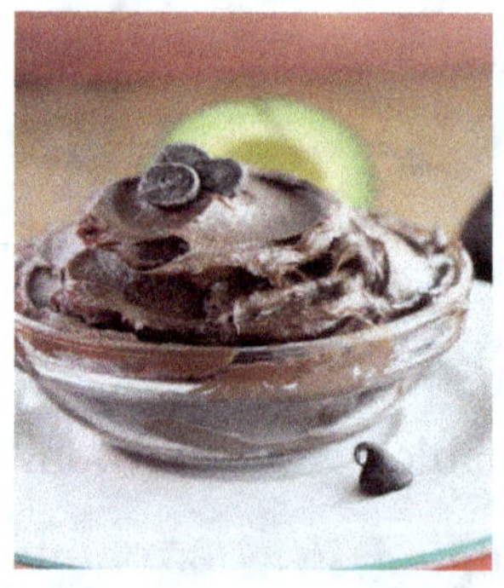

Enjoy this decadent Dark Chocolate Avocado Mousse guilt-free and velvety. This creamy dessert, which is made with the nutrients of ripe avocados and rich dark chocolate, is not only very gratifying but also aids in weight loss.

Prepare to encounter the ideal union of enjoyment and health!

Ingredients:

- 2 ripe avocados
- ¼ cup chocolate powder, unsweetened
- ¼ cup pure maple syrup
- Fresh berries, shaved dark chocolate, or chopped nuts are optional toppings.
- One teaspoon of vanilla flavor.
- One pinch of sea salt.

Instructions:

1. Halve the avocados, scoop out the flesh into a food processor or blender, and discard the pits.

2. Fill the blender or food processor with the cocoa powder, pure maple syrup, vanilla extract, and a dash of sea salt.

3. In order to ensure that all of the components are well incorporated, blend the mixture until it is smooth and creamy.

4. After tasting the mousse, add more maple syrup or cocoa powder to your desire to increase its sweetness or cocoa content.

5. Transfer the mousse to serving bowls or glasses once the preferred flavor and consistency have been reached.

6. Add fresh berries, shaved dark chocolate, or chopped almonds to the mousse's surface for an extra layer of decadence.

7. To help the mousse firm and chill, place it in the refrigerator for at least 30 minutes.

8. To savor the delicious flavors without feeling guilty, serve the dark chocolate avocado mousse cold.

Weight-Loss Benefits

Let's now discuss how this delicious treat can genuinely help you lose weight. Here are some advantages to relish:

1. The avocados, which are the star of this mousse and bring their nutrient-rich goodness to the table, are an excellent source of healthy fats. These luscious fruits are a great source of monounsaturated fats, which can make you feel full and reduce cravings for bad foods.

2. High in Dietary Fiber: Avocados are also a good source of dietary fiber, which is necessary for preserving a healthy digestive tract. Weight loss is facilitated by fiber's role in promoting fullness, regulating hunger, and supporting good digestion.

3. Naturally Sweetened: Instead of using refined sugars, pure maple syrup gives this mousse a hint of natural sweetness. You can indulge while avoiding the detrimental effects of added sugars on your weight loss objectives by choosing a natural sweetener.

5. Filling and Portion Convenient: This mousse is a delightful treat since it combines fiber, dark chocolate flavor, and good fats.

Portion management, which is essential to upholding a balanced approach to weight loss, can be practiced while still indulging in a delectable dessert.

So indulge in a decadent serving of Dark Chocolate Avocado Mousse and take comfort in knowing that you're feeding your body while also gratifying your sweet tooth. Your taste senses will swoon over this rich treat, which will also help you stay on track with your weight loss goals. Good appetite!

Banana Smoothie

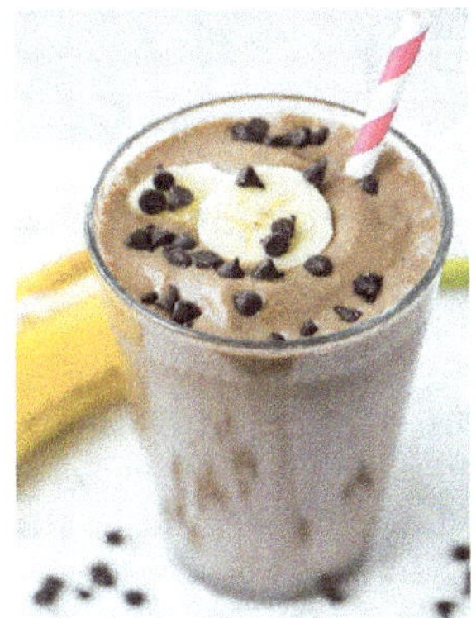

With the help of this invigorating and wholesome Dark Chocolate Banana Smoothie, you can start your day off on a great note.

This smoothie is the ideal blend of enjoyment and health since it is loaded with the benefits of ripe bananas and rich dark chocolate. Prepare to whip up a creamy, chocolatey treat!

Ingredients:

- 2 frozen, peeled bananas that are ripe.
- 1 cup almond milk, unsweetened (or other milk of your choice)

- 2 tablespoons chocolate powder, unsweetened
- 1 teaspoon of raw honey or maple syrup (optional, for extra sweetness)
- A little amount of ice cubes
- ½ teaspoon vanilla extract

Dark chocolate shavings, banana slices, or a dollop of Greek yogurt are available as extra toppings.

Instructions:

1. Blend the frozen bananas, almond milk, chocolate powder, pure maple syrup or honey, vanilla extract, and ice cubes in a blender until smooth.

2. Until they are smooth and creamy, blend the ingredients at high speed. To make sure everything is thoroughly blended, scrape down the sides of the blender as necessary, then reblend.

3. Taste the smoothie and, if necessary, add additional maple syrup or cocoa powder to change the sweetness or level of cocoa.

4. Pour the smoothie into a glass or jar once the ideal flavor and consistency have been attained.

5. Add sliced bananas, Greek yogurt, or shavings of dark chocolate to the smoothie's surface for an extra dash of richness.

6. Enjoy the creamy, chocolatey richness of the Dark Chocolate Banana Smoothie right now!

Weight-Loss Benefits

Let's now discuss the wonderful advantages that this smoothie has for your overall health and weight-loss efforts:

1. Ripe bananas serve as the creamy foundation for this smoothie and add a multitude of nutrients to the mixture. They are a fantastic source of vitamins, minerals, and dietary fiber, all of which promote good digestion, improve muscle function, and offer vital elements for general wellbeing.

2. Gratifying and Energizing: This smoothie combines the indulgent dark chocolate with the naturally sweet bananas to produce a gratifying and energizing delight. Fiber, good fats, and unrefined sugars work together to keep you full, content, and ready for the day.

3. Balanced and Adaptable: The recipe is flexible and may be altered to suit your tastes. To suit your palate while still maintaining a balanced approach to your weight loss goals, you can change the sweetness or cocoa intensity.

4. Quick and Convenient: This smoothie comes up in a flash, making it a practical choice for hectic mornings or as a midday pick-me-up. It's an easy and delectable way to add nutrient-dense ingredients to your diet.

Make a Dark Chocolate Banana Smoothie in your blender to start your day off with a delicious, chocolaty treat. Enjoy this healthy delight while fueling your body and enjoying your favorite flavors. Cheers to a rewarding and healthy adventure!

Yogurt Brownies

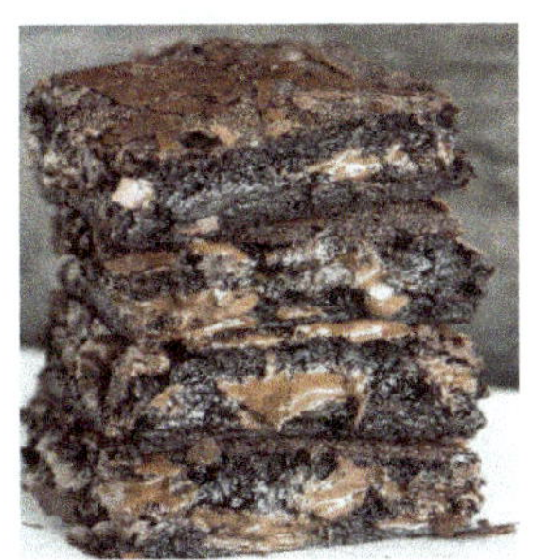

Combine the health advantages of yogurt and dark chocolate and offer portion sizes that may aid in weight loss.

Ingredients:

- One cup of dark chocolate chips
- ½ cup chocolate powder, unsweetened
- ¼ cup coconut oil

- ½ cup Greek yogurt, either low-fat or non-fat

- ½ cup maple syrup or honey

- 2 eggs

- One teaspoon of vanilla extract

- ⅛ teaspoon baking powder

- ½ cup whole wheat flour

- ¼ teaspoon salt

Instructions:

1. Set the oven's temperature to 350°F (175°C). A baking pan should be lined with parchment paper or greased with coconut oil.

2. In a bowl that can be used in the microwave, melt the dark chocolate chips and coconut oil in 30-second intervals while stirring in between. Alternatively, you can constantly whisk them while melting them over low heat on a cooktop.

3. Combine the Greek yogurt, honey (or maple syrup), eggs, and vanilla extract thoroughly in a another mixing dish.

4. Stir the yogurt mixture before adding the chocolate mixture that has been melted into it.

5. Combine the cocoa powder, whole wheat flour, baking soda, and salt in a separate basin.

Stirring until just mixed, gradually add this dry mixture to the wet components. Watch out not to combine too much.

6. Evenly distribute the batter as you pour it onto the prepared baking pan.

7. Bake for approximately 20 to 25 minutes, or until a toothpick inserted into the center of the cake emerges with a few moist crumbs. Avoid overbaking to avoid the brownies drying out.

8. After completely cooling in the pan, cut the brownies into squares or any preferred shapes.

Serving Options

1. Take pleasure in the brownies by themselves as a guilt-free dessert or snack to help you lose weight.

The dark chocolate has a deep, pleasant flavor and may have health advantages.

2. To up the decadence factor, top the brownies with a drizzle of low-fat Greek yogurt and some shaved dark chocolate. The Greek yogurt offers protein and encourages satiety, while the combo adds smoothness and additional chocolate taste.

3. Serve the brownies with a side of fresh berries, like strawberries or raspberries, for a flavorful variation. Berries are a great option for weight loss because they are low in calories and high in fiber.

Weight-Loss Benefits

Greek Yogurt: Greek yogurt is a high-protein food that can help with weight loss. Protein is proven to make people feel more satisfied and helps prevent overeating.

Additionally, Greek yogurt has a lot of calcium, which may help with healthy weight management. Greek yogurt's probiotics support digestive health, which is crucial for general wellbeing.

You can have a gratifying treat while possibly advancing your weight-loss objectives by combining these ingredients in a delectable dessert like Dark Chocolate Yogurt Brownies.

For best results, keep in mind to eat the brownies in moderation and combine them with a healthy diet and frequent exercise.

Gluten-Free Chocolate Cherry Oatmeal Cookies

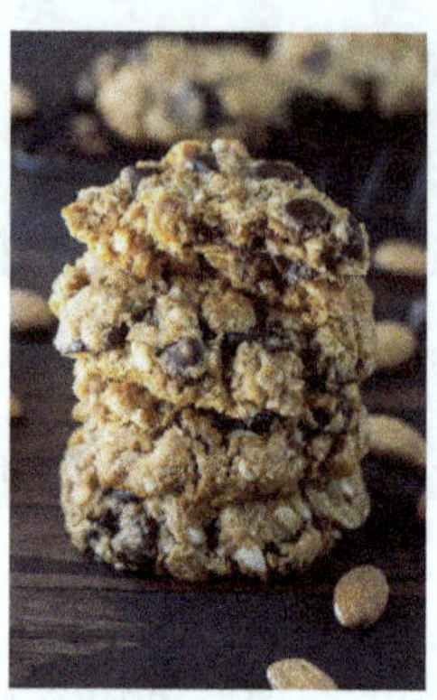

Here is a recipe for gluten-free chocolate cherry oatmeal cookies that makes use of the health benefits of oats, cherries, and gluten-free ingredients and offers serving sizes that can help people lose weight.

Ingredients:

- ½ cup almond flour

- ¼ cup unsweetened cocoa powder

- 1 cup gluten-free rolled oats

- ½ teaspoon baking soda

- ¼ teaspoon of salt

- ¼ cup melted coconut oil

- ¼ cup of honey or maple syrup

- ¼ cup of dark chocolate chips

- ½ cup of chopped dried cherries

- 1 teaspoon of vanilla extract

Instructions:

1. Set the oven's temperature to 350°F (175°C). Use parchment paper to cover a baking sheet.

2. Combine the almond flour, cocoa powder, baking soda, salt, and gluten-free rolled oats in a mixing bowl. To ensure that the dry ingredients are distributed evenly, thoroughly mix.

3. Mix the melted coconut oil, honey (or maple syrup), and vanilla extract thoroughly in a another basin.

4. After combining the wet and dry ingredients, whisk the mixture until a thick dough forms.

5. Evenly distribute the dark chocolate chips and dried cherries throughout the dough by folding them in.

6. Place the dough, in rounded tablespoons, about 2 inches apart on the baking sheet that has been prepared. With the back of a spoon, slightly flatten each cookie.

7. Bake for 10 to 12 minutes, or until the edges start to set. The middle of the cookies might still be a little soft, but as they cool, they will firm up.

8. After the cookies have cooled slightly on the baking sheet, move them to a wire rack to finish cooling.

Serving Options

1. Take pleasure in the cookies as a healthy and filling snack for weight loss. A good dose of fiber, which helps with digestion and makes you feel fuller for longer, is offered by the gluten-free oats.

The addition of cherries and dark chocolate chips gives the cookies a natural sweetness and antioxidants.

2. Combine the cookies with a cup of herbal tea or a glass of unsweetened almond milk for a well-rounded snack option. Without adding too many more calories, this combo helps with desire control and hydration.

3. To make it heartier, sprinkle fresh berries on top of a bowl of low-fat Greek yogurt after crumbling the cookies over it. This results in a low-calorie, high-protein dessert or breakfast choice that is wholesome and filling.

Weight-Loss Benefits:

1. Gluten-Free: These cookies are acceptable for people with gluten sensitivities or for those who follow a gluten-free diet because they are made with gluten-free rolled oats and almond flour.

By avoiding processed foods that frequently include gluten, which in some people may lead to inflammation and weight gain, eating gluten-free can promote weight loss.

2. Cherries: These cookies' dried cherries add a blast of taste and have health advantages. Antioxidants and anti-inflammatory chemicals found in cherries are abundant, which may help to lessen inflammation in the body.
Their inherent sweetness also aids in eliminating the need for processed sugars to sate cravings for sweets.

3. Oats: The addition of gluten-free rolled oats gives the cookies a significant boost in dietary fiber. Fiber encourages satiety, aids in digestion, and can help with weight control by preventing overeating by keeping you pleased and full for extended periods of time.

You can enjoy a treat while possibly advancing your weight-loss objectives by incorporating these gluten-free ingredients, cherries, and oats into delectable Chocolate Cherry Oatmeal Cookies. Keep in mind to consume them in moderation as part of a healthy diet and active way of life.

Whole Grain Chocolate Chip Cookies

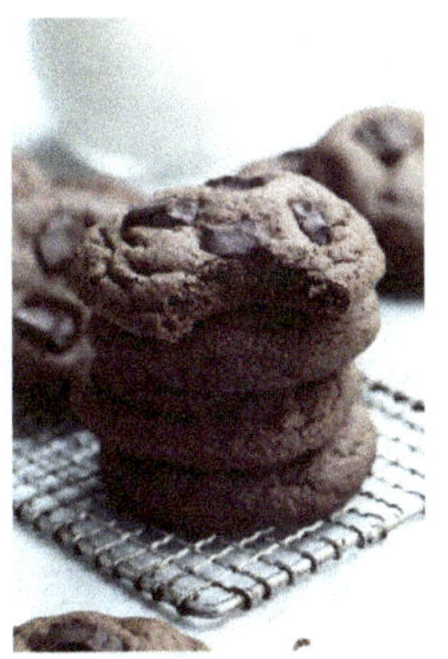

Ingredients:

- 1 cup whole wheat flour

- ½ cup quick-cooking or rolled oats

- ½ teaspoon baking soda

- ½ cup softened unsalted butter

- ¼ teaspoon salt

- ½ cup of brown sugar

- 1 large egg

- ¼ cup granulated sugar

- 1 teaspoon vanilla extract

- ¾ cup chips of dark chocolate

Instructions:

1. Set the oven's temperature to 350°F (175°C). Use parchment paper to cover a baking sheet.

2. Combine the whole wheat flour, oats, baking soda, and salt in a medium basin. Place aside.

3. Combine the softened butter, brown sugar, and granulated sugar in a different mixing dish and beat until frothy. For this step, you can either use a hand mixer or a stand mixer.

4. Beat the butter-sugar mixture well after adding the egg and vanilla essence.

5. Stirring until just combined, add the dry ingredient mixture in small amounts to the wet components. Watch out not to combine too much.

6. Once the dark chocolate chips are included, stir them up thoroughly.

7. Place rounded portions of dough, spaced about 2 inches apart, onto the prepared baking sheet.

8. Bake for 10 to 12 minutes, or until golden brown around the edges. Although the centers of the cookies might still seem a little soft, they will firm up as they cool.

9. Take the baking sheet out of the oven, and after the cookies have cooled on it for a few minutes, move them to a wire rack to finish cooling.

Serving Options

1. Take pleasure in the guilt-free dessert alternative or healthy snack of whole grain chocolate chip cookies. Oats and whole wheat flour offer more fiber and nutrients than regular all-purpose flour.

2. To make a filling and healthy combo, serve the cookies with a cup of green tea or a glass of unsweetened almond milk. These drinks can enhance the cookies' healthy flavor without packing on the calories.

3. To make cookie sandwiches as a special treat, sandwich two cookies together with a layer of natural almond or peanut butter. This increases the amount of protein and good fats, which can increase satiety and aid in weight management.

Weight-Loss Benefits:

1. Whole Grains: Compared to refined grains, the whole grains used in this recipe—whole wheat flour and oats—are high in fiber and have a lower glycemic index.

The presence of fiber makes you feel fuller for longer, which lowers your risk of overeating. Important vitamins, minerals, and antioxidants are also included in whole grains.

You may have a tasty treat while adding more nutritious elements to your diet by using whole grains and dark chocolate chips for your cookies. To assist your weight loss goals, keep in mind to restrict your portion sizes and balance your overall food intake.

No-Bake Dark Chocolate Almond Cookies

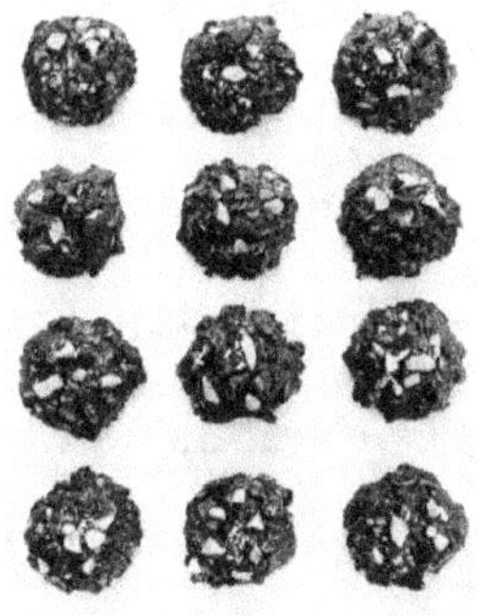

Ingredients:

- 1/4 cup honey or maple syrup
- 1 cup almond butter
- 1 cup rolled oats
- ¼ cup chocolate powder, unsweetened
- ¼ cup chips of dark chocolate
- ¼ cup almonds, chopped
- A dash of salt
- 1 teaspoon of vanilla extract

Instructions:

1. Combine the almond butter, honey (or maple syrup), cocoa powder, dark chocolate chips, chopped almonds, vanilla extract, and salt in a large mixing dish. Stir everything up thoroughly until well-combined.

2. After the ingredients have been thoroughly incorporated, cover the bowl and put it in the fridge for about 30 minutes to let the mixture to firm up.

3. Take the mixture out of the fridge once it has cold. Portion the mixture out using a tablespoon or

cookie scoop, then form it into balls. Put the balls on a dish or baking sheet that has been lined.

4. After the entire mixture has been formed into balls, use the back of a fork to gently press down on each ball to flatten it slightly and shape it into a cookie.

5. Put the cookies back in the fridge and let them chill for another one to two hours, or until they are hard.

6. The cookies are prepared for consumption once they have hardened. For up to a week, keep them in the refrigerator in an airtight container.

Serving Options

1. While trying to lose weight, enjoy the No-Bake Dark Chocolate Almond Cookies as a guilt-free treat or snack. Without baking or additional sugar, these cookies deliver a rich chocolate flavor.

2. For a cozy and low-calorie treat, serve the cookies with a cup of herbal tea or a glass of unsweetened

almond milk. This mixture hydrates the body and may increase a feeling of fullness.

3. Before pressing the cooled cookie dough balls with a fork, roll them in chopped almonds or shredded coconut for extra crunch and nutty flavor. With this modification, the cookies gain texture and nutritional value.

Weight-Loss Benefits:

1. Almonds: Nutrient-rich almonds can help with weight loss. They are a wonderful source of protein, fiber, and healthy fats, all of which help suppress hunger and promote feelings of fullness. Almonds are a good source of calcium, magnesium, and vitamin E, among other necessary vitamins and minerals.

2. Oats: Rolled oats are a complete grain that are high in fiber. By encouraging satiety and assisting with digestion, oats can improve weight loss.

Additionally, oats offer long-lasting energy and are a rich source of essential vitamins and minerals including manganese and phosphorus.

Making these No-Bake Dark Chocolate Almond Cookies will allow you to indulge in a tasty treat while maybe advancing your weight-loss objectives. Always remember to eat them in moderation and include them in a balanced diet and active lifestyle.

Orange Cardamom Chocolate Mousse

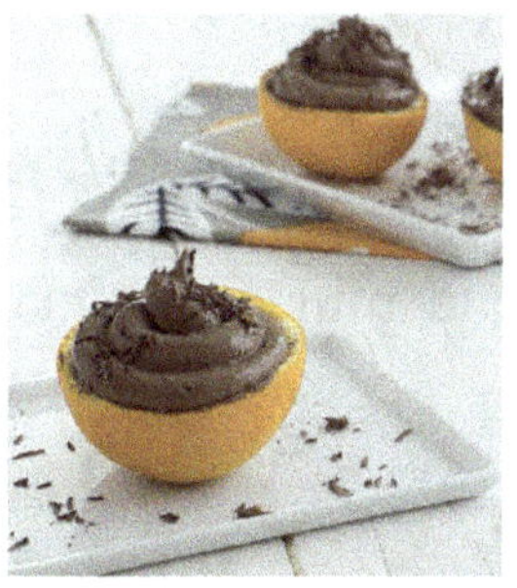

Orange Cardamom Chocolate Mousse combines the health advantages of dark chocolate, orange, and cardamom and offers serving sizes that can be linked to weight loss.

Ingredients:

- 4 ounces of chopped dark chocolate (at least 70% cacao).
- 1 cup almond milk (or other non-dairy milk) without sugar
- 1 tsp. orange zest
- 1/2 tsp. cardamom powder
- 1/4 tsp. vanilla essence
- 1 tbsp. honey or maple syrup (optional; taste before adding)
- Optional garnish of fresh berries

Instructions:

1. Heat the almond milk in a small saucepan over medium heat until it begins to simmer. Get rid of the heat.

2. Stir the heated almond milk with the chopped dark chocolate, then wait a minute to let the chocolate melt. Stir thoroughly and thoroughly until smooth.

3. Include the ground cardamom, vanilla essence, and sweetener (if preferred) along with the orange zest. To thoroughly combine all the flavors, stir well.

4. Pour the mixture into a bowl, cover it with plastic wrap, and chill the mixture for at least two hours, or until the mousse is firm.

5. After the mousse has chilled, take it out of the fridge and give it a quick stir. Pour the mousse into bowls or serving glasses.

6. If you want to add flavor and nutrients, garnish with fresh berries.

Serving Options

1. When trying to lose weight, treat yourself to the luscious but lighter Orange Cardamom Chocolate Mousse. The dark chocolate has a deep, pleasant flavor and may have health advantages.

2. Put some sliced or segmented oranges on the side and serve the mousse with them. Oranges are a

fantastic addition to a diet for losing weight since they are low in calories and high in fiber, vitamin C, and other antioxidants.

3. Sprinkle crumbled almonds or pistachios on top of the mousse for an additional nutritional boost. Nuts are a fantastic source of fiber, protein, and healthy fats that can keep you feeling full for longer and help you control your weight.

Weight-Loss Benefits:

1. Orange: Low in calories and high in vitamin C, fibre, and antioxidants, oranges are a delicious fruit. Vitamin C maintains a strong immune system and may improve fat burning during exercise, which can help with weight management. Oranges' high fibre content encourages fullness and aids in controlling digestion.

2. Cardamom: This spice is well-known for both its flavor and potential health advantages.

Digestion may be facilitated and metabolism may be boosted, both of which are advantageous for weight loss. Additionally, cardamom gives the chocolate mousse a distinct and revitalising flavor.

You may treat yourself to a delectable dessert like Orange Cardamom Chocolate Mousse while possibly achieving your weight-loss objectives by combining these components. For best results, keep in mind to eat in moderation and combine the mousse with a healthy diet and frequent exercise.

CONCLUSION

DARK CHOCOLATE: YOUR DELICIOUS WEIGHT-LOSS FRIEND!

Dark chocolate can be a tasty ally in your quest to lose weight. Explore the delicious and fascinating world of dark chocolate and learn how it might aid in weight loss.

Why limit yourself to just one dark chocolate treat? Let's make it interesting! Pair some wholesome accompaniments with your dark chocolate. Fruits with juicy orange slices or berries are packed with fiber, vitamins, and minerals.

What about nuts, then? Healthy fats and protein are added to the dish with a handful of almonds or walnuts. It's like putting together a dream team of nutrition and flavors to help your weight-loss objectives.

So, my friend, keep in mind that dark chocolate can be your dependable companion as you start your weight-loss journey. Enjoy every attentive bite as you indulge in its antioxidant-rich richness and let it improve your mood.

Just remember that quality counts, so choose products with greater cocoa percentages and stay away from dangerous additives and added sugars. Enjoy that dark chocolate with a smile on your face now that you've adopted a healthy lifestyle and are having fun getting fitter. Because life is too short to not taste achievement, right?

So make dark chocolate your delicious and guilt-free companion on this journey. Cheers to becoming happier and healthier one delectable bite at a time!